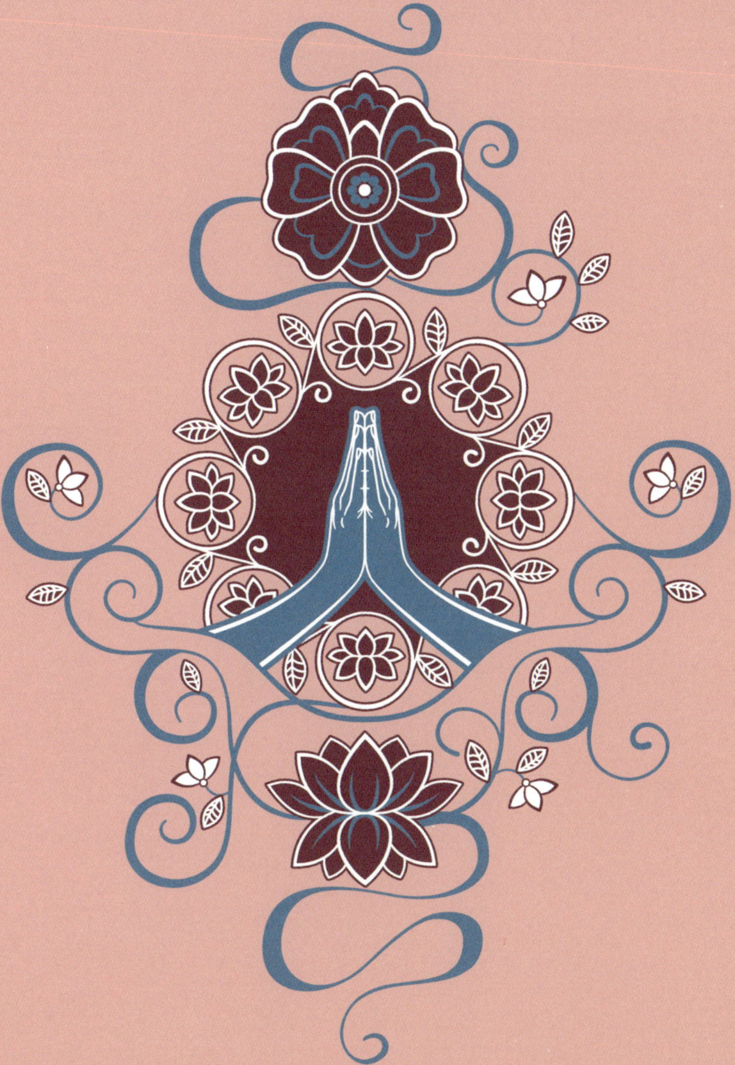

INSIGHTS
A Mandala Journal

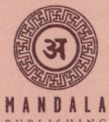

MANDALA
PUBLISHING

www.mandalaearth.com

Tag us on Instagram! @mandalaearth
Copyright © 2019 Mandala Publishing. All rights reserved.
MANUFACTURED IN CHINA
10 9 8 7 6 5 4 3 2 1